10 BEST CANCER FIGHTING FOODS

MARY PAUL

ISBN:9798361801152

DEDICATION

This book is dedicated to God almighty for making this possible and for His direction towads this mouthwatering piece. Also, this book is dedicated to all cancer fighting patients all over the world and to their loved ones that they may find peace within themselves and accept second chances to live through. To my family, for their moral support and love.

CONTENTS

APPLES

Apples include vitamin C, an antioxidant that supports immune system health and prevents the spread of cancer cells. Apples may not only stop tumors, but also aid in the healing process after cancer. Apples have anticancer qualities that could possibly help prevent infections, heart disease, and inflammation.

Numerous photochemical, such as triterpenoids, organic acids, fatty acids, and apple phenolic compounds, are found in apples.

BERRIES

Numerous photochemical and minerals found in blueberries have been shown in studies to have potential anti-cancer properties. According to several studies, consuming blueberries boosts the blood's antioxidant activity and may help prevent DNA damage. Antioxidants are also found in most berries.

Studies demonstrate that these antioxidants shield the body from cell deterioration that may cause skin cancer as well as tumors of the bladder, lung, breast, and esophagus.

Berries are a wonderful source of vitamin C.

Raspberries provide unique advantages for a healthy diet intended to lower the risk of cancer. Their special blend of ellagitannin chemicals and rich dietary fiber has the ability to significantly lower the risk of developing cancer.

CRUCIFEROUS VEGETABLES

In certain epidemiological studies, cruciferous vegetable consumption has been linked to a reduced risk of lung and colorectal cancer, however there is evidence that the impact of cruciferous vegetables on cancer risk in people may depend on genetic polymorphisms.

Cruciferous vegetables and the prevention of cancer have been associated with some degree of research.

Sulforaphane, a compound created from the glucosinolates in broccoli, has been shown in laboratory experiments to inhibit the growth and spread of prostate cancer in a number of different ways.

All cruciferous vegetables include substances known as glucosinolates, which are thought to have anti-cancer properties. After consumption, glucosinolates decompose into isothiocyanates and indoles, which are linked to reduced inflammation and a decreased risk of cancer.

Sulforaphane, a plant ingredient that fights cancer, is particularly abundant in broccoli and has been related to lowering the risks of prostate cancer, breast cancer, colon cancer, and oral malignancies.

Dark green leafy vegetables are rich in fiber, folate, and carotenoids. Examples include mustard greens, lettuce, kale, chicory, spinach, and chard. These vitamins and minerals may offer defense against stomach, lung, skin, oral, throat, and pancreatic cancer. They help protect cells from DNA damage.

Cruciferous vegetables include;

*broccoli

*Cauliflower

*Cabbage

*Kale

* Bok choy

* Arugula

* Brussels sprouts

* Collards

* Watercress

* Radishes

BROCCOLI

Sulforaphane, a plant ingredient that fights cancer and has been associated to lowering the chances of prostate cancer, breast cancer, colon cancer, and oral cancer, is particularly abundant in broccoli.

The malignancies of the prostate, lung, colon, breast, bladder, liver, neck, head, mouth, esophagus, and stomach are the ones that broccoli and its relatives are most effective at preventing.

CAULIFLOWER

Indole-3-carbinol, often known as I3C, is one of these antioxidants and is frequently present in cruciferous vegetables like cabbage, broccoli, and cauliflower. It has been demonstrated to lower both men's and women's chances of developing breast and reproductive cancer.

Although it also exists in orange, green, and purple varieties, white cauliflower is the most popular. Although you might not consider a white vegetable to be a nutritional powerhouse, it really contains substances that prevent the growth of cancer cells and encourage their death while preserving healthy cells.

According to research, those who eat cruciferous vegetables like cauliflower and broccoli have a lower risk of getting cancer. Cauliflower has been eaten since the 12th century or before. It has Middle Eastern roots. Cauliflower is now grown all over the world. One of the main producers is California.

A super food, cauliflower is regarded as having a high nutritional content. Both fiber and vitamins B and C are abundant in it. Additionally, it has significant amounts of glucosinolates and carotenoids, which are antioxidants.

Although both of these substances have anti-cancer properties, interest in glucosinolates has been particularly high.

When cauliflower is cut or chewed, substances known as isothiocyanates (ITCs), which are made of glucosinolates and hinder the growth of cancer, are released.

It is possible to include cauliflower in your diet in a number of different ways, including:

Pureed, steamed, and combined with soups

As an alternative to mashed potatoes, steam and mash

served with a dip as a crudité

grilled or oven-roasted as a side dish (add a touch of parmesan for a truly tasty dish)

Done in floret form and pickled

Use the stem and leaves as well, don't forget. These can be eaten and are also nutritious.

To make soups, blend them.

CABBAGE

It has been demonstrated that cabbage lowers the risk of breast, colon, and rectal cancer. To fully benefit from its cancer-fighting abilities, it should either be consumed completely raw or with very little cooking.

KALE

Another cruciferous vegetable with a high vitamin C and vitamin K content is kale. It is a potent soldier against prostate and colon cancer, lung cancer, and breast cancer, according to research.

According to research, the carotenoids present in dark-green leafy vegetables like kale can work as antioxidants and strengthen the body's natural defenses against free radicals. These safeguards aid in preventing free radicals from damaging DNA, which can result in cancer.

The abundance of rare and powerful photochemical components in **kale** makes it an important food for enhancing human health and lifespan.

This function is accomplished, in part, by shielding our bodies from various biochemical harm and lowering our risk of developing life-threatening chronic illnesses like cancer and heart disease.

The study discovered that steaming maintained the most antioxidants and minerals compared to other cooking techniques, even though raw kale may have the maximum nutritious content, but should be consumed in moderation. It can be used to make salads, with avocados and extra virgin oils inclusive as mixtures.

Bok Choy

According to studies, cruciferous veggies like bok choy help lower your risk of getting cancer. Vitamins C and E, beta-carotene, folate, and selenium are just a few of the cancer-preventing substances found in it.

Like many cruciferous vegetables, raw Bok Choy includes the myrosinase enzyme. Myrosinase can impair thyroid function by obstructing iodine absorption. Cooking turns it off. Moderate amounts of raw bok choy consumption are safe.

This amazing little plant is a great source of fiber, beta-carotene, and vitamins C, K, and A. The cool thing is that both the leaves and the stalks can be eaten. Both calcium and vitamin B6 are abundant in it.

Arugula

Antioxidants, which are substances that can stop or undo cell damage, are abundant in arugula. Glucosinolates are also present in arugula. These organic components, which give arugula its pungent flavor and bitter taste, may shield you from developing some malignancies, such as breast, prostate, lung, and colon cancers.

There is growing proof that arugula may reduce cancer risk. The key phrase here is glucosinolates, a molecule that contains sulfur. Glucosinolates in arugula are converted into indoles, thiocyanates, and isothiocyanates after digestion. According to research, both of these pathways may be used by indole-3-carbinol and the isothiocyanate sulforaphane to prevent cancer.

Eliminate cancer-causing substances and shield cellular DNA from harm

To stop invasion, cause cell death in malignant cells.

You can eat arugula raw or cooked. Arugula can be used raw in salads alone or in conjunction with other lettuces. Due to its strong pepper flavor, it is frequently included in lettuce blends, especially when the arugula is more developed and flavorful. It tastes good on sandwiches too.

BRUSSELS SPROUTS

Reach for the greens; ordinary Brussels sprouts have more health benefits than you might expect.

Ask a group of individuals their thoughts on brussels sprouts, and you'll almost surely get a 50/50 split. Brussel sprouts are a favorite food for certain people, who would eat them every day. Others find it difficult to bear the thought of the soft little cabbages. Even if it can just come down to personal preferences, it is much more likely that individuals who don't like the fiber-rich vegetables have never eaten them properly prepared. Brussels sprouts are no longer dull, tasteless veggies because they are now commonly cooked to a crisp and served with cranberries and syrups. However, despite the fact that cooks have acquired some exquisite skills in the preparation and it's mighty health benefits.

These incredibly absurd-looking vegetables can reduce one's risk of developing a variety of illnesses, from cancer to liver disease. According to research, a substance found in brussels sprouts may help limit tumor growth by obstructing aggressive enzymes known to promote the formation of cancer. The enzymes impair the function of the genes that inhibit cancers and prevent their metastasis. This substance, which is present in Brussels sprouts, enables tumor suppressors to continue to function.

Recipes and how to prepare **Brussels sprouts** delicacy

Oil (to coat pan)

1 bag Brussels sprouts (sliced thin)

¾ cup pesto (homemade or store bought)

1 ½ cups chopped walnuts (or to taste)

Parmesan cheese (if desired)

Preparation

Oil a pan and heat it.
Sliced Brussels sprouts should be sautéed till brilliant green.
Over a low heat, stir in the pesto.
Mix in the toasted walnuts.
Adding parmesan on top is optional.
Warm or cool, enjoy.

COLLARDS

Collard greens are a high source of soluble fiber, vitamin K, and one of the greatest foods for vitamin C. They also contain a variety of nutrients, including sulforaphane and diindolylmethane that have strong anti-cancer potential.

Begin with a thorough soak. Soaking collard greens is the best way to clean them.

Clean the leaves. You ought to notice dirt gathering at the sink's bottom as it drips off the greens.

Leaf drying. With a paper towel or a fresh dishrag, blot the greens dry.

As a side dish, consume them. For more nourishment, add collard greens to a smoothie.

WATERCRESS

Daily consumption of watercress can considerably lessen blood cell DNA damage, which is thought to be a key factor in the emergence of cancer.

It is very significant in the reduction of DNA damage which is the key factor to cancer emergence.

Vitamin C, which is abundant in watercress and supports healthy collagen synthesis as well as your immune system and wound healing, is also good for you. Beta-carotene and other carotenoids, which are considered to be strong antioxidants, are abundant in watercress. It is best to eat it uncooked.

RADISHES

These antioxidants can all aid in preventing cancer. Radish seeds have been shown in studies to kill lung and breast cancer cells. Another study found that the antioxidants in radishes can help provide defense against lung, cervical, breast, prostate, colon, and other malignancies.

Radishes are loaded with fiber, just like any other vegetable. And nothing benefits your digestive system more than fiber.

However, the exact type of fiber that radishes provide is what makes them so excellent for digestion. Lignin is an insoluble fiber that is abundant in radishes. Radishes are difficult for your body to digest, but that specific fiber is still there, soaking up liquids and drawing them into the trash that is created during digestion. And that keeps you regular and ensures that your waste moves gradually through the procedure, avoiding problems like constipation.

Recall how radishes contain vitamin C, which strengthens your immune system? Additionally, radishes have another important health advantage: their high vitamin C concentration may help lower your chance of developing various cancers.

Vitamin C works as an antioxidant to fend off any potential cancer-causing free radicals in your body. It can also prevent cellular damage and reduce inflammation. Additionally, research has indicated that radishes contain various types of antioxidants in addition to vitamin C. They are dispersed throughout the entire plant and are present in the vegetable's roots, sprouts, seeds, and leaves.

These antioxidants can all aid in preventing cancer. Radish seeds have been shown in studies to kill lung and breast cancer cells. According to a different study, radishes' antioxidants can also provide defense against malignancies of the colon, breast, prostate, liver, and lung.

Radishes may or may not offer some kind of protection or risk reduction, but there are many reasons to start eating them more frequently.

CARROTS

Vitamin K, vitamin A, and antioxidants are among the many vital nutrients found in carrots.

Additionally, carrots have a lot of beta-carotene, which gives them their distinctive orange hue.

According to recent research, beta-carotene is essential for immune system support and may shield against several cancers.

According to an analysis, beta-carotene may lower the incidence of breast and prostate cancer.

According to a different analysis, eating more carrots lowers the risk of stomach cancer by 26%. Trusted Source

FATTY FISH

Omega-3 fatty acids, vitamin B, potassium, and other vital elements are abundant in fatty fish, such as salmon, mackerel, and anchovies.

According to one study, persons who consume more freshwater fish in their diets have a 53 percent Trusted Source reduced chance of developing colorectal cancer than those who consume less of it.

The results of additional research

According to a reliable source, consuming fish oil in later age is associated with a much lower chance of developing prostate cancer.

Last but not least, a 68,109-person study found that those who took fish oil supplements at least four times per week had a 63 percent lower risk of developing colon cancer than those who did not.

WALNUTS

All nuts have cancer-fighting qualities, but researchers have focused more of their research on walnuts than other nut varieties.

The body converts pedunculagin, a chemical found in walnuts, into urolithins. Compounds called urolithins bind to estrogen receptors and may help to prevent breast cancer.

Compared to mice given vegetable oil, mice given whole walnuts and walnut oil had higher levels of tumor-suppressing genes, according to a study on animals (Reliable Source).

LEGUMES

Because they include a lot of fiber, legumes may help reduce a person's risk of getting cancer.

Legumes contain a lot of fiber, which may help reduce a person's risk of getting cancer. Examples of legumes include beans, peas, and lentils.

Meta-analysis shows that a higher consumption of legumes is associated with a lower risk of colon cancer, according to 14 studies from a reputable source.

Another study Trusted Source investigates the link between bean fiber consumption and breast cancer risk.

According to the study's findings, those who consumed diets high in bean fiber had a 20% lower risk of breast cancer than those who did not get the recommended amount of fiber each day.

TUMERIC

According to several researches, the curcumin found in turmeric has a number of health advantages, including the ability to combat cancer cells. It may be effective in treating lung, breast, prostate, and colon cancers, according to some laboratory trials. Others claim that curcumin may improve the effectiveness of chemotherapy.

According to research on patients with colorectal cancer, it might decrease the disease's growth. Another study discovered that daily use may reduce the incidence of cancer in those at high risk.

But research on animals or lab-grown cells provides the majority of evidence linking turmeric to cancer. What those studies signify for folks who already have cancer or are attempting to prevent acquiring it is unclear. Ginger had always been considered a miracle root because of its inflammatory properties. But Turmeric, it's close relative is even more beneficial, specifically for it's anti-cancer properties.

zz

TOMATOES

Although, tomatoes are beneficial for your overall health, it is especially useful in fighting prostrate cancer. Fresh tomatoes, as well as products derived from them are rich in Lycopene.

It is this nutrient that makes tomatoes useful for protection against cellular damage and cancer. Whether genetic or not, eating this food cannot be overlooked.

GREEN TEA

If you are already battling cancer , or you simply want to minimize the risk for it, fill up your diet, with these live saving foods . Not only will your body be primed to fight this dreaded disease, but it will also grant you multiple health benefits.

ABOUT THE AUTHOR

Mary Paul is a Nigerian based health practitioner. Her love for humanity has prompted her into this field of being a food health advocate. She has bagged different degrees during the course of her studies to finding diverse remedies to cancer and how it can be minimized'